Table of Contents

What is Hair Loss?.

Anagen Phase.

Catagen (Transitional) Phase.

Telogen (Resting) Phase.

Catch it Early! Knowing the Causes and Signs of Hair Loss.

Male Pattern Baldness.

Female Pattern Baldness.

Other Lesser Known Causes.

Forget Shampoos and Conditioners—The Best ALL NATURAL
Homemade Remedies.

<u>You Are What You Eat—Top Foods for Appearance, Growth and Vitality</u>.

<u>In Review: The Future of Your Hair</u>

Hair Loss Explained

NATURAL Solutions for Hair Loss and Premature Balding

By C.K. Murray

Hair loss.

Nobody wants it. Because losing hair is more than losing hair; hair is more than appearance. It's not important, it's *everything*. Hair represents beauty and grace. In men, it's a testament of masculinity and power. It imbues us with confidence, giving us flair and faith, creating an impression of who we are and what we want. In women, hair does much the same—if not more. It shines, it glimmers, it flows and falls. Which is why losing it can be so devastating. It doesn't matter who you are, watching a once-lush head of hair thin and fade before your eyes… is *disheartening* to say the least.

But there's a solution!

If you're losing hair, you're not losing 'you.' You can still reclaim your scalp and bring back the better days. The number one thing to remember is simple: know the facts, make the change. If you have a firm understanding of the methods, the *all-natural* methods, you stand more than a fighting chance. In fact, having the right methods in your arsenal can make a world of difference. It can be the difference between embarrassment and pride. Between hiding your head or sharing your looks with the world.

Tired of what you're seeing? Let's not waste any more time, here's what you need to know…

What is Hair Loss?

You've seen it, but what does it mean? Are you destined for baldness? Are you going to have a thick head of hair for a long time? What is normal and what indicates an issue?

Truth be told, we all lose hair. Out of the near 150,00 hairs on our heads, some 100 to 125 of them fall out each and every day. Hair is all over our bodies, ranging from the top of our head to our sometimes hobbit-like feet. Hair can turn up in small patches or thick growths, everywhere on the body but our palms and our feet soles. When hair follicles produce new hair cells, those hair cells are pushed outward, eventually reaching visible hair. The protein, keratin, is what is produced in those hair follicles, and by the time hair is visible, we are looking at *dead* keratin.

Most people grow hair at a rate of 6 inches per year, or half an inch per month. At any one time, 85-90% of the hair on your scalp is growing. Of course, these numbers can quickly change. When observing the life cycle of a given hair, it is important to consider all of the factors. Firstly, what is your race? Hair color, texture, and curliness vary. Caucasian hair is a combination of other races, Asian hair is the thickest, with a straight hair follicle and hair shaft.

African hair, by contrast, has curved follicles with a curly hair shaft. Asian and African hair are invariably black, while Caucasian hair can be anywhere from black to blonde. In blondes, the hair itself is finer, but the number of hairs is greater.

Of course, race is but a part of the equation. Factors such as age, health, weather exposure and personal hygiene can all go far in determining the life of your hairs. And when it comes to that life cycle, there are three phases to consider:

Anagen Phase

This is the phase in which your hair is growing. For healthy heads of hair, 85-95% of your hair is in this phase at all times. This stages lasts anywhere from a couple years to over half a decade. The metabolism of the hair root is peaked during this stage, causing quick growth. However, because the hair cells are dividing so quickly, the hair is more sensitive than normal to diseases and other conditions.

Catagen (Transitional) Phase

This is the shortest phase and lasts just a few weeks. The growth of new hair declines and the root actually shrinks to almost a third of its original size.

Telogen (Resting) Phase

This phase lasts roughly a quarter to a third of a year. Hair falls out during this period, whether because it has reached its limit, or because a new hair is growing, and thus pushing it out. On a healthy head of hair, the lost hairs are simply replaced as the anagen phase begins again. However, when this balance is upset, the number of growing hairs on your head may plummet far below the norm of 85%...

Catch it Early! Knowing the Causes and Signs of Hair Loss

Why do we lose hair? Is it because we're too careless? Do we expose our hair too much to the elements? To heat and cold? Is it because we're too rough, combing and brushing and yanking our hair this way and that? Gelling it, drying it, shampooing and dyeing it?

Does hair give up because we've destroyed it? With all the chemicals in our products?

What if we're too *gentle*? What if we never gave our hair the exposure it needed? What if from day one, we coddled it and protected it, never allowing our locks to develop the strength they deserved?

What causes hair loss? Truth be told, there are *many* causes, and the majority of them are under our control. Of course, some people say otherwise. Some people will tell you that it's out of your control. That losing hair is going to happen, no matter what you do. They'll point to your loved ones, to your relatives. They'll say that it 'runs in your family,' that it's going to happen—no matter what—and that you might as well get used to it.

Well they're wrong. While there is no denying a genetic component to certain types of hair loss, this doesn't mean that you can't significantly affect your hair health. Fortunately, there are many things, easy things, that you can do. *Unfortunately*, many people have no idea what to do. This is because many people have no idea what even causes their hair loss.

Whether man or woman, guy or girl, elder, teenager, young adult, or middle-ager—it's never too late to act. So don't worry. Don't fret. Get yourself in the game and start putting your knowledge to use. If you're finding more and more hair on your brush or comb, in the shower drain or on your pillow—and less and less on your head—the time is *now* to act!

A typical hair grows from its follicle at about 1/2 inch per month. Each hair grows for 2-6 years, remains for a period, and then falls out. After falling out, a new hair begins growing from the follicle. What we consider baldness is the *absence* of those new hairs.

Let's go over the causes:

Male Pattern Baldness

This is probably the most common. This is the one that people like to talk about when they say simply, "You're going to lose it." Fortunately, male pattern baldness can be recognized early. That means that you can begin *treating* it early. If you're not sure if you're experiencing male pattern hair loss, simply consider what you're going through.

When it comes to male pattern baldness, there are various stages, some obviously more noticeable than others. According to the American Hair Loss Association, male pattern baldness makes up 95% of hair loss in men, and by age 35, two-thirds of men will have noticeable hair loss, with 85% of men over 50 having significantly thinned hair. Almost 1/4th of men begin losing hair before their 21st birthday.

Also known as androgenetic alopecia, male pattern baldness is caused by a sensitivity to dihydrotestosterone (DHT). Dihydrotestosterone (DHT) is a by-product of testosterone. This means that DHT occurs naturally with the presence of testosterone; it is created through the help of important enzymes, and causes hair follicles to shrink, becoming frail and falling out. Although it is sometimes true that balding men may have more testosterone than their non-balding counterparts, the truth is more specific: DHT-*sensitive* men are more susceptible to hair loss. A man can have a lot of testosterone, but if his hair follicles are not as susceptible to DHT, a man with far less testosterone may bald more.

Male pattern baldness is usually noticeable once the hairline starts receding and the crown begins thinning in Stage 2. In more advanced stages, this balding and thinning causes a horseshoe pattern of hair seen in Stage 7. For many men who reach this stage early on, the appearance can be nothing sort of debilitating. Fortunately, affecting your body's DHT levels is not only possible but *probable* with the right strategies.

Female Pattern Baldness

Androgenetic alopecia also affects women. Although hair is not lost in the same style or fashion as in males, females can certainly experience considerable hair loss. According to the Academy of Dermatology, forty percent of women have visible hair loss by the time they are age 40.

The reasons for female pattern baldness are not as well understood as they are in men. That said, hormonal levels are also believed a factor in women. Aside from merely losing hair due to the attrition of age, women may lose hair following menopause. This happens because the balance of male hormones, androgens, changes in women. Menopause may cause women to have a noticeable increase in facial hair, but decrease in head hair. Experts also point to a genetic component, but lack a firm understanding of its basis.

For women who are experiencing androgenetic alopecia, the signs are usually quite telling. Firstly, the thinning pattern is different than it is in men. In women, the hair gets thinner mostly on the top and crown of your head, with a widening mid-line as you can see in the above pictures. Unlike in men, the front hairline remains intact and the hair loss *rarely* gets to a point of total baldness. Even so, substantial hair loss can and does occur.

Other Lesser Known Causes

You might be shaking your head. What if you don't have male pattern or female pattern baldness, yet are still losing hair? What if hair is coming out in sudden patches, or in strange irregular patterns? Well, if this is the case, you've got to consider other factors.

According to the American Academy of Dermatology, there are

numerous hair loss 'disorders.' They are:

- **Cicatricial alopecia:** This one is rare and can happen even if you're a perfectly healthy human. Basically, it eradicates the hair follicles themselves, leaving an unpleasant scarring. In the end, this scarring actually covers the area of the former follicle. As a result, your hair will not grow back—unless, of course, the inflammation is treated.

- **Alopecia areata:** An alleged autoimmune disorder in which the body attacks itself. This results in smooth and round patches of hair loss. In most cases, these individuals are in good health and experience regrowth. However, the growth is slow.

- **Central centrifugal cicatricial alopecia:** Like "cicatricial alopecia," this one leads to hair loss and scarring. Unlike normal cicatricial alopecia, this one afflicts mostly women of African descent. It radiates from the center of the scalp, causing the scalp to become smooth and shiny. The spots of hair loss may burn, tingle, itch and scar. If scarring occurs, the likelihood of regrowth is diminished..

Stress and Diet

Stress is a known cause of hair loss. Traumatic events such as death or injury can cause hair loss, as can chronic exposure to the stress hormone cortisol. Childbirth is another stressful event that can cause hair loss. Women will notice this as a result of plummeting estrogen, but they will gain their hair back in no time later. Another stage of hair loss in women is menopause, as mentioned earlier. This will also regrow with time. Through cortisol optimization, both men and women can mitigate the negative effects of stress.

In addition to traditional mental and physical stress, the stress of dieting is also powerful. A lot of people actually lose hair when they have lost around 20lbs or more. This happens as the body adjusts biochemically, and the hair typically returns by half a year at the latest.

But this isn't always the case. If you hair doesn't return after losing weight, it might have to do with what's in your diet. Research shows that Vitamin A causes hair loss when ingested excessively through vitamins or supplements. It's also important to optimize Vitamin D. If you are optimizing your vitamin levels, don't forget your protein. Among vegetarians especially, protein deficiency is problematic. Hair growth slows and hair loss may occur as a result of too little protein. Vegetarians can remedy this by adding more nuts, seeds, and beans to their diet.

Beans are also good for iron intake. Not to mention you can pair them up with other iron rich foods such as certain cereals, lentils, soybeans, pumpkin seeds, spinach, oysters, clams, and liver. As long as you are ingesting enough vitamins, nutrients, and protein, any hair loss is likely *not* the result of diet.

Disease

There are numerous medical conditions that cause an individual to lose hair. More than 25 diseases are known to affect hair loss, with the most common being anemia and thyroid issues. If treated, the hair loss can usually be prevented or even reversed. In addition to such diseases, major illnesses have also been linked to hair loss. Having a very invasive surgery, struggling with an extended high fever, or contracting a bad infection or flu can all cause hair loss. Treatments for major illnesses such as cancer can also cause hair loss. Ringworm of the scalp can even lead to hair loss among children. In most cases, this disease or medically-indicated balding is called *telogen effluvium.*

A final type of hair loss is called *trichotillomania.* This actually refers to a psychological disorder in which people are compelled to pull out their own hair. They may even pull out eyelashes or eyebrows. Anywhere that hair grows on their body may become areas to target. The causes for this compulsion are still largely unknown.

Medicines

A final cause of hair loss is medication. As you know, there are a million different medications out there, each with its host of possible side effects. If you are experiencing hair loss and believe it's medicine-related, check the list. Medications that cause hair loss include:

- Vitamin A supplements (especially high doses)

- Birth control pills

- Medications for depression, arthritis, heart problems, gout and hypertension

- Blood thinners

- Anabolic steroids

Although hair loss is not probable in the use of these medications, it is certainly possible. When noticing hair loss, be sure to note how long you've taken the medication and if you've started doing anything else that may be contributing. Physicians will typically prescribe something else, if they can, that minimizes the risk.

Of course, hair loss is not only caused by medications, diets, diseases and disorders. If you find that your head is thinning and your hairline receding, it's time to act. Before doing anything drastic, consider your showering regimen. Think about the shampoos and conditioners you may be using, and do one, simple thing: Get rid of them!

Forget Shampoos and Conditioners—The Best ALL NATURAL Homemade Remedies

If you didn't know by now, most shampoos *aren't* your friend. In fact, many of the products we use on our head contain potentially dangerous chemicals. Not to mention, many of the methods we use for hair care are also hazardous. One hundred or so shampoos have already been found to have a chemically modified, cancer-causing chemical. And if this isn't bad enough, many now argue that shampoos and conditions are simply unnecessary.

Shampoos and other hair products can be pricey. They can contain carcinogens, pesticides, hormone modulators and toxins that affect reproductive capability. They can also deprive your scalp of its natural oil lubricant, sebum. When sebum is repeatedly stripped from your scalp, your body begins to depend upon the shampoo. In other words, your scalp forgets how to produce its own sebum, meaning that you have to spend more and more money just to achieve levels that were once normal. It becomes a pricey, counterproductive cycle of hair products and beauty concerns.

Of course, the product you choose is just part of the problem. How you apply it and use it can also be a huge issue. A lot of us like to use bleaching products that cause the hair to break and thin. Too many gels, dyes, relaxers and hair sprays leads to hair that is brittle. Limiting use is especially important among women who observe excessive broken hairs.

We also have to be mindful of the way we dry our hair. Blow dryers can be our best friends, if used in moderation. But when misused, they're a disaster. The high heat can actually boil water in our hair shafts, exacerbating breakage. Not to mention, devices like flat and curling irons are highly dangerous. They are *especially* good at killing hair.

And if this isn't bad enough, a lot of us are weakening our heavenly heads with accessories. Rubber bands, clips and hairpins are typical culprits. When choosing rubber bands, it's best to choose scrunchies that can be located around the scalp to reduce stress in one area. Hairpins should have smoother, ball-tipped surfaces, and hair *clips* should have rubber paddings where they touch the hair. Over time, ponytails, cornrows and braids may degrade the quality of the hair. A perpetual pull on the hair that causes hair loss is known as *traction alopecia*.

A lot of people also make the mistake of washing, drying and combing the hair improperly. Here are some cardinal rules to remember when it comes to these practices:

Don't rub wet hair with a towel; massage it or let it just hang and dry

Limit brush and combing of wet hair

Do not exceed 100 strokes in shampooing, combing or brushing a day

Hair is more elastic wet than dry, so be careful. Unless you're of African descent, wet hair will be more susceptible to breakage. Of course, these are merely tips for caring for your hair. The most important thing to know is what you put in that hair. Instead of opting for expensive, convoluted shampoos and hair products, go the All-Natural route…

Again, shampoo can be very problematic, especially for those with waves or curls. By cutting back on shampoos, not only do we give hair back its natural body and fullness, but we also cure it of dangerous toxins. Drying sulfates like ammonium lauryl sulfate and sodium laureth sulfate are in most shampoos. If we leave these sulfates out of our hair, we promote a head of hair that is less frizzy and more cooperative.

Here are some amazing homemade remedies that can immediately replace your overpriced shampoos and conditioners. Many of them constitute powerful health hacks that can be applied in all areas of your life:

Coconut Oil

Haven't heard of this one?

Then wake up! Coconut oil is not only a superfood, it's a wonderful cosmetic product. Great for skin, hair, and just about anywhere you decide to rub it (except your eyes, don't put it in your eyes). Jokes aside, coconut oil is incredible. It can promote strong proteins, seal in moisture, fight bacteria and fungi, infuse vitamins and nutrients, and boost blood circulation.

Firstly, coconut oil contains lauric acid, a fatty acid that binds well to hair proteins and protects hair roots. It is actually more effective at preventing hair loss than many other oils such as mineral and sunflower oils found in most hair care products. Not to mention, coconut oil application is a sustainable practice. It penetrates the hair instead of merely sitting on it and coming off during rinsing. It even has the power to reduce DHT levels, an important factor in androgenetic alopecia.

When it comes to sealing in moisture, coconut oil is an all-star. Because it penetrates so easily, it actually conditions your hair from the inside-out. This helps to keep your hair safe and sound, even in the face of environmental factors such as heat and pollution. And speaking of pollution, coconut oil helps to ward off lice, dandruff and other irritants—all thanks to its antibacterial and antifungal capabilities. Coconut oil also contains lots of vitamins E & K, as well as iron. This means that your hair gets the nutrients it needs for shine and softness. Finally, coconut oil is great for blood circulation. By massaging your hair with coconut oil, you stimulate blood flow, which then keeps your hair going strong. In other words, rub in that oil and give your head the rub-and-love it deserves and needs!

But be careful. Not all coconut oils are created equally. It's best to use a product that is unrefined, organic Virgin Coconut Oil (VCO). Nutiva and Dr.Bronner's make great products of this kind. Once you have this oil in your hands, it's time to follow suit:

Firstly, rewarm the jar in warm water to bring the coconut oil from its solid state to a more runny, easily applicable oil state. Next, warm your own hair with warm water. Make sure your hair is nice and damp and use one tbsp. of coconut oil. Apply directly to the roots of your hair by using your fingertips to massage in. Feel free to use as much as you want, though it might take some experimenting to get the right level.

Make sure to massage for several minutes, taking your time and treating your hair tenderly. Afterwards, wait roughly half an hour before thoroughly washing out. You will not need a conditioner for this process.

If you'd like, you can also leave in coconut oil overnight or for extended periods. Research shows that leaving in small amounts for 14 hours yields the best results. Of course, this may vary depending upon your hair and the amount applied. Starting out, do not be alarmed if a couple hairs fall out when initially rubbing in the oil. This is natural, and your hair will strengthen and grow back quicker as a result of coconut oil application. And also, be sure to eat coconut oil! It's a tremendous complement to any meal. There are numerous coconut oil recipes.

Vinegar

Another topical treatment is vinegar. The best is Apple Cider

Vinegar or white vinegar, which are great ways to affect dandruff. Vinegar removes dying skin cells and also acts as a fungicide. In order to do this, you need to have a half cup of warm water, a half cup of ACV or white vinegar, and an empty cup. Mix the warm water and vinegar in the cup and pour it over your hair, scrubbing it around and then rinsing with water. You should wait roughly half a day before taking a normal shower. Feel free to vinegar rinse once a week or every two weeks in addition to your other more frequent treatments.

Rosemary

Rosemary is a very powerful herb, especially for hair growth and vitality. The herb has antioxidant powers that are good for hair growth, as well as sulfur and silica. These two constituents help reverse hair loss, and rosemary is also great for increasing circulation and clearing hair follicles.

When making the mix, be sure to use two drops of rosemary essential oil in two tablespoons of an oil like coconut, olive, jojoba or avocado oil. Massage it in the hair and be sure to leave it in for roughly half an hour before shampooing as usual. Also feel free to use rosemary water as a treatment. Steep several sprigs in a couple cups of hot water for 5 minutes or so. You can also boil the dried form of the herb. After heating it, allow it to cool and then strain. You can use this rosemary water for rinsing after your shower.

Both of these approaches can be used several times per week.

Lemon Juice

Lemons have always been great for hair health. They contain tons of vitamin C and vitamins B1, B2, B3, B5, B6, B12, folic acid, and other nutrients. Not to mention, they are loaded with antioxidants. In addition to spurring hair growth, lemon juice will get your hair shiny and dandruff free. It stimulates circulation, but used too often, may cause your hair to lighten. To prepare lemon juice, mix one part lemon juice with two parts of coconut or olive oil. Put it on your hair and scalp, leaving for 45 minutes, then wash it out. This can be done once or twice a week.

Cayenne pepper

Cayenne pepper is great for promoting hair growth and reducing loss. It contains capsaicin, which gives it its hotness. When applied to the scalp, cayenne pepper stimulates blood flow and gets the nerves firing on full. Simply mix one tbsp. of pepper powder with two tbsps. of coconut oil. Apply it to areas of the scalp where thinning is most obvious. Wash off with cool water after 15 minutes.

Egg Gel

This home remedy may sound a little odd, but it's actually renowned for its positive effects. See, eggs naturally contain high amounts of protein, which is obviously important for keeping your hair strong. Eggs also contain zinc, iron, sulphur, selenium, phosphorous and iodine. When you make this gel, use the white of one or two eggs and add 1 or 2 teaspoons of coconut oil and honey. You've really got to mix this one well until it's a nice smooth paste. Leave in your hair for 20 minutes before washing off with cool water.

Peppercorn Paste

Black peppercorns are central to ayurvedic medicine. They make the hair soft and lustrous, keeping it hydrated and healthy. To make this mix, simply blend a couple teaspoons of peppercorns with a half cup of lemon or lime juice. Apply this paste to your roots and cover your head with a warm towel to trap in the penetration. After about half an hour, take off. Black peppercorns are rich in essential oils and a great natural way to keep your hair looking young and feeling lively.

Onion Juice

Onion juice is a smelly and eye-watering solution to thinning hair. It stimulates your hair to grow due to its rich sulphur content. Sulphur is known to produce collagen tissues, which assist in hair regrowth. Red onions or shallots will work perfectly. Simply grab 2-4 onions, grate them and squeeze out the juice, and massage them into the scalp. You should leave the juice in your hair for an hour before washing out normally.

You can also take 4-5 chopped onions and throw them in boiling water. Once boiled for 10 minutes or so, let the water cool and wash with it. This works best if you don't wash your hair again for at least a day. If you can't stand the smell or have places to be and people to see, you can cut that time accordingly.

Mint Tonic

Mint has plenty of powerful effects and can make your hair smell amazing. Simply mix several tablespoons of dried mints in 1 cup of water with a half cup of vinegar. Simmer for about 5 minutes before allowing to cool. Then strain and work it into your hair, allowing 10 minutes or so for it to soak in before washing out.

Avocado hair mask

Avocado is great for treating hair that is lacking in necessary vitamins and nutrients. Avocados are rich in vitamins B and E, which spur growth and repair damage. To get these benefits, mash an avocado and massage into hair. It's really that easy! Then, wrap a towel on your head or a shower cap. Allow at least 10 minutes before washing out as normal.

Alright, so now you have a better idea of some very nifty techniques. They all feature items that you can acquire readily, and do not require a great investment of time, effort, or money. If you're looking to enjoy all-natural hair remedies, the aforementioned treatments are perfect! However, maybe they're not enough. Applying the right topical treatments for hair care is only part of the issue.

Your success also depends largely on your lifestyle. And if you aren't eating the right foods, you're shooting yourself in the foot (and head!)

You Are What You Eat—Top Foods for Appearance, Growth and Vitality

Everybody knows that eating healthy is important. Still, this doesn't mean everybody *does* it. The problem with eating healthy is that it takes work; sometimes real work. And not everybody likes real work.

Which is why you'll be happy to know that there is a shortcut. Superfoods (and super drinks) are all around us. They don't require a large quantity and they don't make us feel 'weird.' They're normal, natural foods, and if you can master them, you'll slowly but surely improve your hair.

Let's not waste any more time. Let's get down the vitamins and foods you need. They are:

Beetroot Juice

What is beetroot juice? Firstly, beetroot is a vegetable that you can juice or put through a blender then strainer. It is a veritable goldmine of goodies, filled with protein, calcium, iron, potassium, magnesium, carotenoids, vitamins B and C, phosphorus and silica. It should be consumed regularly, and if you don't like the taste, feel free to combine with many other juices and concoctions. Cucumbers, carrots, and other vegetables are great complements. If you're seeking various fruit and vegetable blends, start a juice cleanse diet today.

Omega-3s

Omega-3 fatty acids are essential nutrients for continued health. Aside from making your hair shiny and strong, omega-3s do a host of other things. They help control blood clotting, promote new cell membranes in the brain, protect the heart, and fight inflammation. Basically, omega-3 fatty acids are great for overall health, and because our body does not produce them naturally, they *must* come from foods in our diets. This is why so many people are deficient in this category.

When eating omega-3 rich foods, there are essentially two types of omega-3s. There is the kind found in vegetable oils, seeds and nuts and the kind found in fatty fish. The first kind can be consumed through soybean, canola and flaxseed oils as well as in walnuts. It can also be enjoyed in leafy greens such as kale, brussel sprouts, salad greens and spinach. The second kind of mega-3s must be obtained from fatty fish. These fish include salmon, sardines, mackerel and even tuna, among others. It is important to get at least one rich serving of omega-3s per day. Fish oil supplements can also be an alternative if your diet simply won't cooperate.

Proteins

The average person requires between one and a half and two and a half ounces of protein per day. Compromised immune systems are especially needy. If you want to feel good and look good too, protein will get you there. Because over ¾ of human hair is comprised of the protein keratin, consuming protein in your diet is paramount.

Basically, the science is this: our bodies require amino acids for protein synthesis. Our bodies makes 11 of these essential amino acids, but the other 9 must come from our diets. If we fail to get a balance of all 20 for an extended period, the follicles may actually lose their ability to produce hair fiber. In rare cases, severe and sudden balding will occur.

When it comes to getting the proteins you need, think simple. You want a balance, so make sure to eat meat, fish, eggs, dairy products, and poultry. In terms of meat and poultry, opt for round steak, ground beef (90% lean), boneless pork chops, and boneless and skinless chicken breasts. For fish, opt for yellowfin tuna, halibut, salmon, and tilapia. For dairy products, cottage cheese, thick greek yogurt, swiss cheese, and 2% milk are high-protein choices.

Of course, don't go overboard. Don't focus on protein to the exclusion of other essential dietary elements. The important thing, as always, is to balance your foods. This may seem like a daunting task, as there are so many different food groups to consider. However, a good rule of thumb is to adopt the DASH diet. It's not only great for your heart, but has been shown year after year to benefit virtually every major area of human health.

Iron

Iron is amazing. But too many people are getting too little. When we talk of iron deficiency, we are not simply referring to a condition that causes weakness and compromised bodily functions. We are quite literally referring to what could be a life-changing, or ending, condition. For this reason, getting enough iron is critical, and very important for boosting hair health. It's no wonder then, that researchers have linked alopecia, severe hair loss and brittle hair to iron deficiency.

Although the average adult only needs 1-1.5mg of iron per day, this small amount is often hard to come by. The difficulty lies in the fact that iron is not always easily absorbed. In fact, one-third of the world's population is believed to be deficient, as only a fraction (`18%) of the iron we eat is absorbed. Those at risk for iron deficiency include babies who don't get enough breast milk or formula, teenage girls, menstruating women, people with poor diets, vegetarians and vegans, over-trained athletes, people with diseases like cancer and kidney disease, and regular blood donors.

The role of iron is crucial. It facilitates oxygen transport in haemoglobin, a complex protein that comprises roughly two thirds of the body's iron. Iron also makes up myoglobin, a protein that stores oxygen in muscle cells and gives muscles their red hue. Enzymes, that drive cellular functions, are also fueled by iron. Not to mention your immune system! This is the reason that people feel weak and lethargic when low on iron.

So eat iron! Get it in your red meat like liver, get it in iron-fortified cereals, in green leafy vegetables like kale and spinach, in turkey, beans and even dried fruits.

Vitamins

The final category to worry about is that of vitamins. All of the vitamins play a significant role in energizing our bodies and brains, and keeping our normal functions intact. Firstly, there's vitamin A. This vitamin keeps hair shiny by moisturizing and preventing drying. Vitamin A allows the hair to thicken naturally, and can be found in liver, egg yolks, milk, spinach, mangoes, sweet potatoes and carrots.

Another important vitamin is vitamin B12. This one facilitates absorption of iron. It is found in eggs and milk like vitamin A, but can also be obtained from cheese, yogurt and whey powder. Another vitamin in the B-family is vitamin B71:1 or Biotin. This vitamin increases the production of cells, fatty acids within those cells, and aids other processes related to amino acids and fats. If you are deficient in Biotin, getting enough can have drastic effects. It has been shown to dramatically increase growth rate, straighten hair and increase volume. If you're lacking this crucial vitamin, you need eggs, yeast, raspberries, almonds, walnuts, bananas, and cauliflower.

Another important vitamin for hair is the famous vitamin C. As you probably already know, vitamin C is found easily in oranges. It is great for preventing premature greying and can keep your hair from drying out. If you need more, try to enjoy other fruits such as mandarins, lemons and strawberries.

Once you've upped your C-levels, feel free to get the final vitamin, vitamin E. This one is also great for moisturizing, and can keep your scalp healthy through improved blood circulation. To get enough E, consume foods such as fish, milk, peanuts, dried herbs, sunflower seeds and almonds.

And there you have it. Eating right and improving your hair health does not have to be hard. If all of this sounds like too much work, think of it this way: balance. I've said it already and I'll continue to say it. Life is about balance. If you pour yourself into one food group exclusively, your body will simply lack what it needs. Many times, our taste buds and 'cravings' tell us what we're lacking. But if they don't, simply take some time.

Think about what your daily diet is like. Do you get enough fruits? Are you a person that hates vegetables? Are there ways you can prepare vegetables or include them in other meals that would make them more enjoyable? Are you getting enough red meats? While many people are scared into thinking too much red meat will kill them, there is certainly a need to get *some*.

Are you somebody that doesn't like milk? Have you tried goat's milk and other animal milks? Have you tried different kinds of fish? What about beans and nuts? Have you tried to diversity your meals?

At the end of the day, what's the verdict—Do you eat for health or for *convenience*?

In Review: The Future of Your Hair

As you know by now—if you didn't already—hair is complex. Saying that somebody is going to lose hair or not lose hair without knowing the details is simply foolish. Every time you look at your own head or somebody else's head, don't assume that because that person has 'better' hair, that he or she is somehow genetically superior.

There are numerous factors that affect hair strength, growth, volume, and appearance. There are numerous factors that affect scalp health and overall body and brain health. If your hair is thinning, receding or falling out in strange patterns, consider your behaviors. Do you shower too frequently, use hazardous shampoos and conditioners, not eat like you should, dry, rub and brush your hair too much? What's your deal? What's your habit?

Is it your attitude? Is a stressful existence killing your follicles and weakening your shafts? Do you ever find yourself literally pulling out your hair? Do you feel like it at times?

The bottom line is this: consider your lifestyle. Opt for natural methods, and avoid assembly line formulas that pump out false promises and faulty products.

Give your hair the life it needs and wants. *Au Naturale*

A Special Note:

Thank you for reading *"Hair Loss Explained: NATURAL Solutions for Hair Loss and Premature Balding."* If you enjoyed reading this book and would like to be included on an email list for when similar content is available, feel free:

SUBSCRIBE

As always, thank you for reading.

And may you continue to live healthily and happily.

Sincerely,

C.K. Murray

Other works by C.K. Murray:

1. *Mindfulness Explained: The Mindful Solution to Stress, Depression, and Chronic Unhappiness*

2. *Emotional Intelligence Explained: How to*

Master Emotional Intelligence and Unlock Your True Ability

3. *The Confidence Cure: Your Definitive Guide to Overcoming Low Self-Esteem, Learning Self-Love and Living Happily*

4. *Let Love Flourish: The Secret to Finding Your Kindred Heart*

5. *Body Language Explained: How to Master the Power of the Unconscious*

6. *A Reason to Smile: Finding Happiness in Life's Little Moments*

7. *Health Hacks: 46 Hacks to Improve Your Mood, Boost Your Performance, and Guarantee a*

Longer, Healthier, More Vibrant Life

8.   *Depression, Drugs, & the Bottomless Pit: How I found my light amid the dark*

9.   *The Stress Fallacy: Why Everything You Know Is WRONG*

10.*Master Mind: Unleashing the Infinite Power of the Latent Brain*

11.*Sex Science: 21 SIZZLING Secrets That Will Transform Your Bedroom into a Sauna*

12. *Sex Secrets: How to Conquer the Power of Sexual Attraction*

13. *Master of the Game: A Modern Male's Guide to Sexual Conquest*

14. *Persuasion Explained: How to Use Your Inner Eye to Influence Others*

15. *Deep Sleep: 32 Proven Tips for Deeper, Longer, More Rejuvenating Sleep*

16. *The Blood Pressure Diet: 30 Recipes Proven for*

Lowering Blood Pressure, Losing Weight, and Controlling Hypertension

17. *Coconut Oil Cooking: 30 Delicious and Easy Coconut Oil Recipes Proven to Increase Weight Loss and Improve Overall Health*

18. *High Blood Pressure Explained: Natural, Effective, Drug-Free Treatment for the "Silent Killer"*

19. *The Wonders of Water: How H2O Can Transform Your Life*

20.*INFUSION: 30 Delicious and Easy Fruit Infused Water Recipes for Weight Loss, Detox, and Vitality*

21.*The Ultimate Juice Cleanse: 25 Select Juicing Recipes to Optimize Weight Loss, Detox and Longevity*

22.*ADHD Explained: Natural, Effective, Drug-Free Treatment For Your Child*

23.*Confidence Explained: A Quick Guide to the Powerful Effects of the Confident and Open Mind*

24. *How to Help an Alcoholic: Coping with Alcoholism and Substance Abuse*

25. *Vitamin D Explained: The Incredible, Healing Powers of Sunlight*

26. *Last Call: Understanding and Treating the Alcoholic Brain (A Personal and Practical Guide)*

27. *Hooked: Life Lessons of an Alcoholic and Addict (How to Beat it Before it Beats YOU)*

28. *Neuro-Linguistic Programming Explained: Your Definitive Guide to NLP Mastery*

29. *Natural Weight Loss: PROVEN Strategies for Healthy Weight Loss & Accelerated Metabolism*